Understanding Diabetes

Improve Your Diabetic Lifestyle

Prevention & Cure For Diabetic Living

By : Gala Publication

2

Published By :

Gala Publication

© Copyright 2015 – Gala Publication

ISBN-13: **978-1519685544**
ISBN-10: **1519685548**

Table of Contents

Chapter 1:
What is Diabetes?

Diabetes, often referred to by doctors as diabetes mellitus, describes a group of metabolic diseases in which the person has high blood glucose (blood sugar), either because insulin production is inadequate, or because the body's cells do not respond properly to insulin, or both. Patients with high blood sugar will typically experience polyuria (frequent urination), they will become increasingly thirsty (polydipsia) and hungry (polyphagia).

Diabetes can strike anyone, from any walk of life.

And it does – in numbers that are dramatically increasing. In the last decade, the cases of people living with diabetes jumped almost 50 percent – to more than 29 million Americans.

Worldwide, it afflicts more than 380 million people. And the World Health Organization estimates that by 2030, that number of people living with diabetes will more than double.

Today, diabetes takes more lives than AIDS and breast cancer combined -- claiming the life of 1 American every 3 minutes. It is a leading cause of blindness, kidney failure, amputations, heart failure and stroke. Living with diabetes places an enormous emotional, physical and financial burden on the entire family. Annually, diabetes costs the American public more than $245 billion.

Just what is diabetes?

To answer that, you first need to understand the role of insulin in your body.

When you eat, your body turns food into sugars, or glucose. At that point, your pancreas is supposed to release insulin.

Insulin serves as a "key" to open your cells, to allow the glucose to enter -- and allow you to use the glucose for energy.

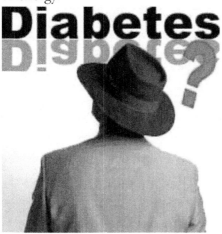

But with diabetes, this system does not work.

Several major things can go wrong – causing the onset of diabetes. Type 1 and type 2 diabetes are the most common forms of the disease, but there are also other kinds, such as gestational diabetes, which occurs during pregnancy, as well as other forms.

There are three types of diabetes:

TYPE 1

In type 1 diabetes, the pancreas is unable to produce any insulin, the hormone that controls blood sugar levels. Type 1 diabetes typically appears in childhood or adolescence, but its onset is also possible in adulthood. When it develops later in life, type 1 diabetes can be mistaken initially for type 2 diabetes. Correctly diagnosed, it is known as latent autoimmune diabetes of adulthood.

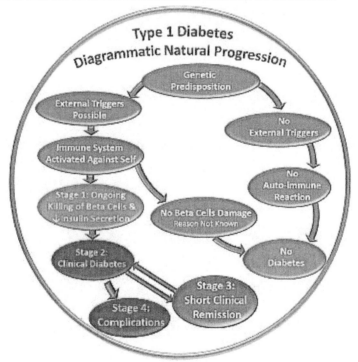

Insulin production becomes inadequate for the control of blood glucose levels due to the gradual destruction of beta cells in the pancreas. This destruction progresses without notice over time until the mass of these cells decreases to the extent that the amount of insulin produced is insufficient.

TYPE 2

Insulin resistance is usually the precursor to type 2 diabetes - a condition in which more insulin than usual is needed for glucose to enter cells. Insulin resistance in the liver results in more glucose production while resistance in peripheral tissues means glucose uptake is impaired. Obesity can lead to insulin resistance - often the precursor to the development of type 2 diabetes.

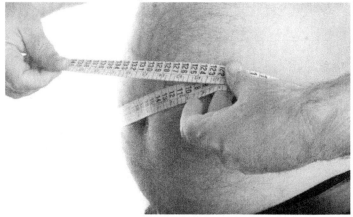

The impairment stimulates the pancreas to make more insulin but eventually the pancreas is unable to make enough to prevent blood sugar levels from rising too high.

Genetics plays a part in type 2 diabetes - relatives of people with the disease are at a higher risk, and the prevalence of the condition is higher in particular among Native Americans, Hispanic and Asian people.

Obesity and weight gain are important factors that lead to insulin resistance and type 2 diabetes, with genetics, diet, exercise and lifestyle all playing a part. Body fat has hormonal effects on the effect of insulin and glucose metabolism.

Once type 2 diabetes has been diagnosed, health care providers can help patients with a program of education and monitoring, including how to spot the signs of hypoglycemia, hyperglycemia and   other diabetic complications.

As with other forms of diabetes, nutrition and physical activity and exercise are important elements of the lifestyle management of the condition.

Chapter 2:
Symptoms

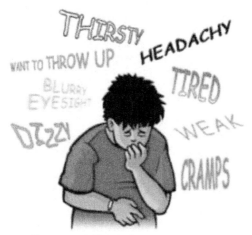

Common Symptoms

Both types of diabetes have some of the same telltale warning signs.

Hunger and fatigue. Your body converts the food you eat into glucose that your cells use for energy. But your cells need insulin to bring the glucose in.

If your body doesn't make enough or any insulin, or if your cells resist the insulin your body makes, the glucose can't get into them and you have no energy. This can make you more hungry and tired than usual.

Peeing more often and being thirstier. The average person usually has to pee between four and seven times in 24 hours, but people with diabetes may go a lot more.

Why? Normally your body reabsorbs glucose as it passes through your kidneys. But when diabetes pushes your blood sugar up, your body may not be able to bring it all back in. It will try to get rid of the extra by making more urine, and that takes fluids.

You'll have to go more often. You might pee out more, too. Because you're peeing so much, you can get very thirsty. When you drink more, you'll also pee more.

Dry mouth and itchy skin. Because your body is using fluids to make pee, there's less moisture for other things. You could get dehydrated, and your mouth may feel dry. Dry skin can make you itchy.

Blurred vision. Changing fluid levels in your body could make the lenses in your eyes swell up. They change shape and lose their ability to focus.

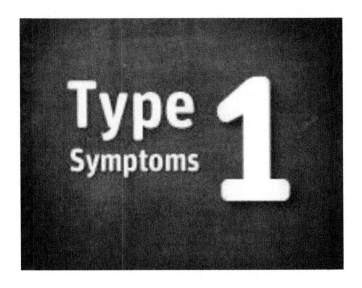

The 4Ts - symptoms of type 1 diabetes
What are the 4Ts?

The 4Ts of type 1 diabetes are:

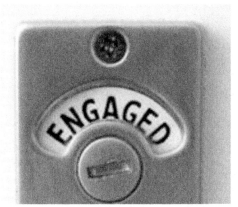

Toilet

The need to go to the toilet more frequently is called polyuria.

Needing to visit the toilet more often than usual, going during the night when you usually don't or having very short breaks between going to the toilet are all part of one of the main symptoms of type 1 diabetes.

If a child starts to regularly wet the bed, having not wet the bed for some time, it could also indicate a sign of diabetes.

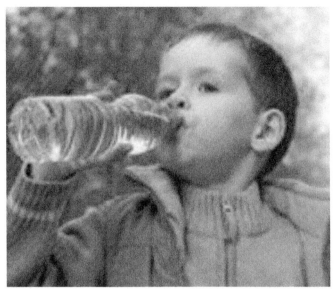

Thirsty

Excessive thirst which results in increased fluid intake.

We all get thirsty from time but thirst can be a symptom of type 1 diabetes. Some signs of unusual thirst may include:

- Regularly getting up to drink during the night
- Drinking a full glass or bottle of liquid and still being very thirsty
- Having only gaps between bouts of thirst

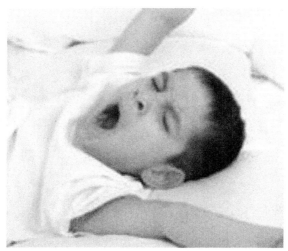

Tired

Feeling extra tired, lethargic or having fatigue

When the body lacks insulin, as happens in type 1 diabetes, cells of the body cannot take in glucose from the blood for energy which can leave the body tired and unnourished.

Tiredness in type 1 diabetes may be spotted if someone who is usually active starts finding physical activity particularly difficult to carry out.

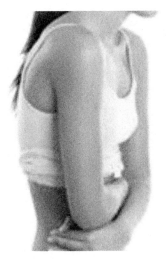

Thinner

An increased appetite that is not satisfied by eating more

A lack of insulin means the body cannot get enough glucose from the blood into cells and so the body starts to break down fat and muscle into ketones to use as an alternative source of energy.

A symptom of type 1 diabetes is therefore exaggerated and/or unexplained loss of body weight.

Symptoms of Type 2 Diabetes

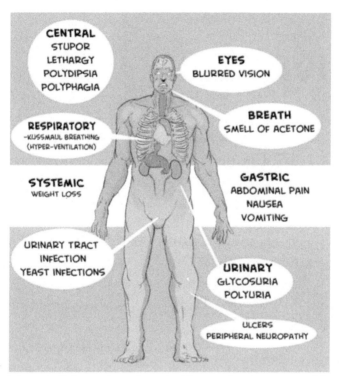

Type 2 diabetes is a chronic disease that can cause blood sugar (glucose) to be higher than normal. Many people do not feel symptoms with type 2 diabetes. However, there are some common symptoms that it is important to be aware of. Most symptoms of type 2 diabetes occur when blood sugar levels are abnormally high.

The most common symptoms of type 2 diabetes include:

- excessive thirst
- frequent or increased urination, especially at night
- excessive hunger
- fatigue
- blurry vision
- sores or cuts that won't heal

If you experience any of these symptoms on a regular basis, talk to your doctor. They may recommend that you be tested for diabetes, which is performed with a basic blood draw. Routine diabetes screening normally starts at age 45. However, it might start earlier if you are:

- overweight
- sedentary
- affected by high blood pressure, now or when you were pregnant
- from a family with a history of type 2 diabetes
- from an ethnic background that has a higher risk of type 2 diabetes
- at higher risk due to high blood pressure, low good cholesterol levels, or high triglyceride levels

Common Symptoms of Type 2 Diabetes

If you have diabetes, it can help to understand how your blood sugar levels affect the way you feel. Most common symptoms of diabetes are caused by elevated glucose levels.

Frequent or Increased Urination

Elevated glucose levels force fluids from your cells. This increases the amount of fluid delivered to the kidneys.

This makes you need to urinate more. It may also eventually make you dehydrated.

Thirst
As your tissues become dehydrated, you will become thirsty. Increased thirst is another common diabetes symptom. The more you urinate, the more you need to drink, and vice versa.

Fatigue
Feeling worn down is another common symptom of diabetes. Glucose is normally one of the body's main sources of energy. When cells cannot absorb sugar, you can become fatigued or feel exhausted.

Blurred Vision
In the short term, high glucose levels can cause a swelling of the lens in the eye. This leads to blurry vision. Getting your blood sugar under control can help correct vision problems. If blood sugar levels remain high for a long time, other eye problems can occur.

Recurring Infections and Sores
Elevated glucose levels may make it harder for your body to heal. Therefore, injuries like cuts and sores stay open longer. This makes them more susceptible to infection.

Sometimes, people don't notice that they have high blood sugar levels because they don't feel any symptoms.

High blood sugars can lead to long term problems, such as a higher risk for heart disease, foot problems, nerve damage, eye diseases, and kidney disease. People with diabetes are also at risk for serious bladder infections. In people without diabetes, bladder infections are usually painful. However, diabetics may not have that sensation of pain with urination. The infection may not be detected until it has spread to the kidneys.

Part 3 of 3: Emergency Symptoms

Emergency Symptoms of Type 2 Diabetes

As stated, high blood sugar causes long-term damage to the body. However, low blood sugar, called hypoglycemia, can be a medical emergency. Hypoglycemia occurs when there are dangerously low levels of blood sugar. For people with type 2 diabetes, only those people who are on medications that increase the body's insulin levels are at risk for low blood sugar.

Symptoms of hypoglycemia include:

- shaking
- dizziness
- hunger
- headache
- sweating
- trouble thinking
- irritability or moodiness
- rapid heartbeat

If you are on medicines that incease the amount of insulin in your body, be sure you know how to treat low blood sugar.

Chapter 3:
Causes

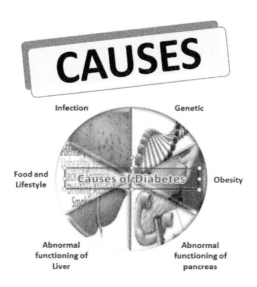

What causes type 1 diabetes?

Type 1 diabetes is caused by a lack of insulin due to the destruction of insulin-producing beta cells in the pancreas. In type 1 diabetes—an autoimmune disease—the body's immune system attacks and destroys the beta cells. Normally, the immune system protects the body from infection by identifying and destroying bacteria, viruses, and other potentially harmful foreign substances. But in autoimmune diseases, the immune system attacks the body's own cells. In type 1 diabetes, beta cell destruction may take place over several years, but symptoms of the disease usually develop over a short period of time.

Type 1 diabetes typically occurs in children and young adults, though it can appear at any age. In the past, type 1 diabetes was called juvenile diabetes or insulin-dependent diabetes mellitus.

Latent autoimmune diabetes in adults (LADA) may be a slowly developing kind of type 1 diabetes. Diagnosis usually occurs after age 30. In LADA, as in type 1 diabetes, the body's immune system destroys the beta cells. At the time of diagnosis, people with LADA may still produce their own insulin, but eventually most will need insulin shots or an insulin pump to control blood glucose levels.

Genetic Susceptibility

Heredity plays an important part in determining who is likely to develop type 1 diabetes. Genes are passed down from biological parent to child. Genes carry instructions for making proteins that are needed for the body's cells to function. Many genes, as well as interactions among genes, are thought to influence susceptibility to and protection from type 1 diabetes. The key genes may vary in different population groups. Variations in genes that affect more than 1 percent of a population group are called gene variants.

Certain gene variants that carry instructions for

making proteins called human leukocyte antigens (HLAs) on white blood cells are linked to the risk of developing type 1 diabetes. The proteins produced by HLA genes help determine whether the immune system recognizes a cell as part of the body or as foreign material. Some combinations of HLA gene variants predict that a person will be at higher risk for type 1 diabetes, while other combinations are protective or have no effect on risk.

While HLA genes are the major risk genes for type 1 diabetes, many additional risk genes or gene regions have been found. Not only can these genes help identify people at risk for type 1 diabetes, but they also provide important clues to help scientists better understand how the disease develops and identify potential targets for therapy and prevention.

Genetic testing can show what types of HLA genes a person carries and can reveal other genes linked to diabetes. However, most genetic testing is done in a research setting and is not yet available to individuals. Scientists are studying how the results of genetic testing can be used to improve type 1 diabetes prevention or treatment.

Autoimmune Destruction of Beta Cells

In type 1 diabetes, white blood cells called T cells attack and destroy beta cells. The process begins well before diabetes symptoms appear and continues after diagnosis. Often, type 1 diabetes is not diagnosed until most beta cells have already been destroyed. At this point, a person needs daily insulin treatment to survive. Finding ways to modify or stop this autoimmune process and preserve beta cell function is a major focus of current scientific research.

Recent research suggests insulin itself may be a key trigger of the immune attack on beta cells. The immune systems of people who are susceptible to developing type 1 diabetes respond to insulin as if it were a foreign substance, or antigen. To combat antigens, the body makes proteins called antibodies. Antibodies to insulin and other proteins produced by beta cells are found in people with type 1 diabetes. Researchers test for these antibodies to help identify people at increased risk of developing the disease. Testing the types and levels of antibodies in the blood can help determine whether a person has type 1 diabetes, LADA, or another type of diabetes.

Environmental Factors

Environmental factors, such as foods, viruses, and toxins, may play a role in the development of type 1 diabetes, but the exact nature of their role has not been determined. Some theories suggest that environmental factors trigger the autoimmune destruction of beta cells in people with a genetic susceptibility to diabetes. Other theories suggest that environmental factors play an ongoing role in diabetes, even after diagnosis.

Viruses and infections. A virus cannot cause diabetes on its own, but people are sometimes diagnosed with type 1 diabetes during or after a viral infection, suggesting a link between the two. Also, the onset of type 1 diabetes occurs more frequently during the winter when viral infections are more common. Viruses possibly associated with type 1 diabetes include coxsackievirus B, cytomegalovirus, adenovirus, rubella, and mumps. Scientists have described several ways these viruses may damage or destroy beta cells or possibly trigger an autoimmune response in susceptible people. For example, anti-islet antibodies have been found in patients with congenital rubella syndrome, and cytomegalovirus has been associated with significant beta cell damage and acute pancreatitis—inflammation of the pancreas. Scientists are trying to identify a virus that can cause type 1 diabetes so that a vaccine might be developed to prevent the disease.

Infant feeding practices. Some studies have suggested that dietary factors may raise or lower the risk of developing type 1 diabetes. For example, breastfed infants and infants receiving vitamin D supplements may have a reduced risk of developing type 1 diabetes, while early exposure to cow's milk and cereal proteins may increase risk. More research is needed to clarify how infant nutrition affects the risk for type 1 diabetes.

What causes type 2 diabetes?

Type 2 diabetes—the most common form of diabetes—is caused by a combination of factors, including insulin resistance, a condition in which the body's muscle, fat, and liver cells do not use insulin effectively. Type 2 diabetes develops when the body can no longer produce enough insulin to compensate for the impaired ability to use insulin. Symptoms of type 2 diabetes may develop gradually and can be subtle; some people with type 2 diabetes remain undiagnosed for years.

Type 2 diabetes develops most often in middle-aged and older people who are also overweight or obese. The disease, once rare in youth, is becoming more common in overweight and obese children and adolescents. Scientists think genetic susceptibility and environmental factors are the most likely triggers of type 2 diabetes.

Genetic Susceptibility

Genes play a significant part in susceptibility to type 2 diabetes. Having certain genes or combinations of genes may increase or decrease a person's risk for developing the disease. The role of genes is suggested by the high rate of type 2 diabetes in families and identical twins and wide variations in diabetes prevalence by ethnicity. Type 2 diabetes occurs more frequently in African Americans, Alaska Natives, American Indians, Hispanics/Latinos, and some Asian Americans, Native Hawaiians, and Pacific Islander Americans than it does in non-Hispanic whites.

Recent studies have combined genetic data from large numbers of people, accelerating the pace of gene discovery. Though scientists have now identified many gene variants that increase susceptibility to type 2 diabetes, the majority have yet to be discovered. The known genes appear to affect insulin production rather than insulin resistance. Researchers are working to identify additional gene variants and to learn how they interact with one another and with environmental factors to cause diabetes.

Studies have shown that variants of the *TCF7L2* gene increase susceptibility to type 2 diabetes. For people who inherit two copies of the variants, the risk of developing type 2 diabetes is about 80 percent higher than for those who do not carry the gene variant.[1] However, even in those with the variant, diet and physical activity leading to weight loss help delay diabetes, according to the Diabetes Prevention Program (DPP), a major clinical trial involving people at high risk.

Genes can also increase the risk of diabetes by increasing a person's tendency to become overweight or obese. One theory, known as the "thrifty gene" hypothesis, suggests certain genes increase the efficiency of metabolism to extract energy from food and store the energy for later use. This survival trait was advantageous for populations whose food supplies were scarce or unpredictable and could help keep people alive during famine. In modern times, however, when high-calorie foods are plentiful, such a trait can promote obesity and type 2 diabetes.

Obesity and Physical Inactivity

Physical inactivity and obesity are strongly associated with the development of type 2 diabetes. People who are genetically susceptible to type 2 diabetes are more vulnerable when these risk factors are present.

An imbalance between caloric intake and physical activity can lead to obesity, which causes insulin resistance and is common in people with type 2 diabetes. Central obesity, in which a person has excess abdominal fat, is a major risk factor not only for insulin resistance and type 2 diabetes but also for heart and blood vessel disease, also called cardiovascular disease (CVD). This excess "belly fat" produces hormones and other substances that can cause harmful, chronic effects in the body such as damage to blood vessels.

The DPP and other studies show that millions of people can lower their risk for type 2 diabetes by making lifestyle changes and losing weight. The DPP proved that people with prediabetes—at high risk of developing type 2 diabetes—could sharply lower their risk by losing weight through regular physical activity and a diet low in fat and calories. In 2009, a follow-up study of DPP participants—the Diabetes Prevention Program Outcomes Study (DPPOS)—showed that the benefits of weight loss lasted for at least 10 years after the original study began.[2]

Read more about the DPP, funded under National Institutes of Health (NIH) clinical trial number NCT00004992, and the DPPOS, funded under NIH clinical trial number NCT00038727 in Diabetes Prevention Program.

Insulin Resistance

Insulin resistance is a common condition in people who are overweight or obese, have excess abdominal fat, and are not physically active. Muscle, fat, and liver cells stop responding properly to insulin, forcing the pancreas to compensate by producing extra insulin. As long as beta cells are able to produce enough insulin, blood glucose levels stay in the normal range. But when insulin production falters because of beta cell dysfunction, glucose levels rise, leading to prediabetes or diabetes.

Abnormal Glucose Production by the Liver

In some people with diabetes, an abnormal increase in glucose production by the liver also contributes to high blood glucose levels. Normally, the pancreas releases the hormone glucagon when blood glucose and insulin levels are low. Glucagon stimulates the liver to produce glucose and release it into the bloodstream. But when blood glucose and insulin levels are high after a meal, glucagon levels drop, and the liver stores excess glucose for later, when it is needed. For reasons not completely understood, in many people with diabetes, glucagon levels stay higher than needed. High glucagon levels cause the liver to produce unneeded glucose, which contributes to high blood glucose levels. Metformin, the most commonly used drug to treat type 2 diabetes, reduces glucose production by the liver.

The Roles of Insulin and Glucagon in Normal Blood Glucose Regulation

A healthy person's body keeps blood glucose levels in a normal range through several complex mechanisms. Insulin and glucagon, two hormones made in the pancreas, help regulate blood glucose levels:

- Insulin, made by beta cells, lowers elevated blood glucose levels.
- Glucagon, made by alpha cells, raises low blood glucose levels.

When blood glucose levels rise after a meal, the pancreas releases insulin into the blood.

- Insulin helps muscle, fat, and liver cells absorb glucose from the bloodstream, lowering blood glucose levels.
- Insulin stimulates the liver and muscle tissue to store excess glucose. The stored form of glucose is called glycogen.
- Insulin also lowers blood glucose levels by reducing glucose production in the liver.

When blood glucose levels drop overnight or due to a skipped meal or heavy exercise, the pancreas releases glucagon into the blood.

- Glucagon signals the liver and muscle tissue to break down glycogen into glucose, which enters

the bloodstream and raises blood glucose levels.
- If the body needs more glucose, glucagon stimulates the liver to make glucose from amino acids.

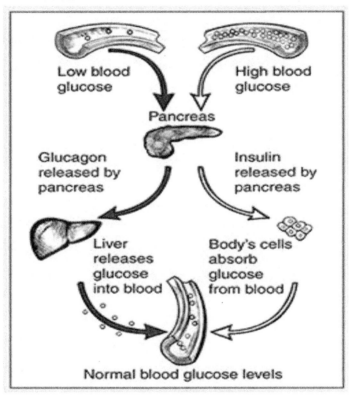

Insulin and glucagon help regulate blood glucose levels.

Metabolic Syndrome

Metabolic syndrome, also called insulin resistance syndrome, refers to a group of conditions common in people with insulin resistance, including

- higher than normal blood glucose levels
- increased waist size due to excess abdominal fat
- high blood pressure
- abnormal levels of cholesterol and triglycerides in the blood

People with metabolic syndrome have an increased risk of developing type 2 diabetes and CVD. Many studies have found that lifestyle changes, such as being physically active and losing excess weight, are the best ways to reverse metabolic syndrome, improve the body's response to insulin, and reduce risk for type 2 diabetes and CVD.

Cell Signaling and Regulation

Cells communicate through a complex network of molecular signaling pathways. For example, on cell surfaces, insulin receptor molecules capture, or bind, insulin molecules circulating in the bloodstream. This interaction between insulin and its receptor prompts the biochemical signals that enable the cells to absorb glucose from the blood and use it for energy.

Problems in cell signaling systems can set off a chain reaction that leads to diabetes or other diseases. Many studies have focused on how insulin signals cells to communicate and regulate action. Researchers have identified proteins and pathways that transmit the insulin signal and have mapped interactions between insulin and body tissues, including the way insulin helps the liver control blood glucose levels. Researchers have also found that key signals also come from fat cells, which produce substances that cause inflammation and insulin resistance. This work holds the key to combating insulin resistance and diabetes. As scientists learn more about cell signaling systems involved in glucose regulation, they will have more opportunities to develop effective treatments.

Beta Cell Dysfunction

Scientists think beta cell dysfunction is a key contributor to type 2 diabetes. Beta cell impairment can cause inadequate or abnormal patterns of insulin release. Also, beta cells may be damaged by high blood glucose itself, a condition called glucose toxicity.

Scientists have not determined the causes of beta cell dysfunction in most cases. Single gene defects lead to specific forms of diabetes called maturity-onset diabetes of the young (MODY). The genes involved regulate insulin production in the beta cells. Although these forms of diabetes are rare, they provide clues as to how beta cell function may be affected by key regulatory factors. Other gene variants are involved in determining the number and function of beta cells. But these variants account for only a small percentage of type 2 diabetes cases. Malnutrition early in life is also being investigated as a cause of beta cell dysfunction. The metabolic environment of the developing fetus may also create a predisposition for diabetes later in life.

Risk Factors for Type 2 Diabetes

People who develop type 2 diabetes are more likely to have the following characteristics:

- age 45 or older
- overweight or obese
- physically inactive
- parent or sibling with diabetes
- family background that is African American, Alaska Native, American Indian, Asian American, Hispanic/Latino, or Pacific Islander American
- history of giving birth to a baby weighing more than 9 pounds
- history of gestational diabetes
- high blood pressure—140/90 or above—or being treated for high blood pressure
- high-density lipoprotein (HDL), or good, cholesterol below 35 milligrams per deciliter (mg/dL), or a triglyceride level above 250 mg/dL
- polycystic ovary syndrome, also called PCOS
- predieteacosis nigricans, a condition associated with insulin resistance, characterized by a dark, velvety rash around the neck or armpits
- history of CVD

The American Diabetes Association (ADA) recommends that testing to detect prediabetes and type 2 diabetes be considered in adults who are overweight or obese and have one or more additional risk factors for diabetes. In adults without these risk factors, testing should begin at age 45.

Chapter 4:
Living With Diabetes

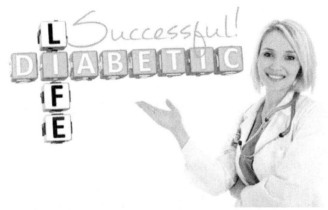

Being diagnosed with diabetes, or knowing someone who is diagnosed with the condition, may throw up many questions about how it fits into your daily life, from how it makes you feel to managing diabetes at work, or whilst you are driving. This section provides information about how diabetes can fit around you and your life.

Being diagnosed with diabetes and living with diabetes can sometimes feel overwhelming – this is quite normal. In this section of the website you can find out more about how diabetes may affect your emotions and how you feel.

Your emotions

One of the most difficult things to come to terms with is that diabetes is for life. In the weeks and months after being diagnosed with diabetes, emotions are often pushed to one side as you try to get to grips with new treatments and changing your lifestyle. Everyone reacts differently when they hear the news. You may be overwhelmed, shocked, afraid, angry and anxious. Some people go through a stage very similar to mourning –as though they are grieving for lost health Some people hide these feelings, but that doesn't necessarily mean that they are coping without difficulty. Over time it is likely that you will become more confident in your ability to cope with everyday activities, and the initial turmoil you may have felt should start to fade.

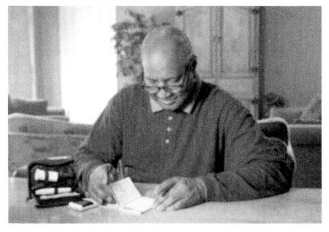

Your healthcare team

Your healthcare team is there to give you emotional support, reassurance and help you to build your confidence in coping with diabetes. If you, your family, or friends are concerned about any aspect of diabetes, your healthcare team would rather know about it. If the worry is groundless, then you can be reassured. If it has some cause then action can be taken.

You can also get a lot of support and encouragement from other people with diabetes – Diabetes UK Local Groups and Care events give you the change to hear how others cope in similar situations. People respond in different ways to being diagnosed with diabetes – some to the extent that they feel like hiding it from everyone. You may feel embarrassed and uncertain about how they will react, but letting people know can mean that you receive more support and understanding. Family and friends may be among the first people you tell, and like most people they probably know little about diabetes – but are keen to know more.If you live alone, telling your neighbours about your diabetes may make you feel safer, especially if you are older or at risk of having hypos. A simple explanation to your housemate may help their understanding too.If you are taking part in sport or physical activity it is sensible to tell the person who is leading the activity in case any problems arise.

Giving up smoking

If you are a smoker and have been diagnosed with diabetes, giving up the habit is one of the most positive things you can do to both improve your health and reduce your risks of the long-term complications associated with the condition.

Everyone risks damaging their health through smoking a cigarette, pipe or cigar, but for people with diabetes the risk may be even greater.

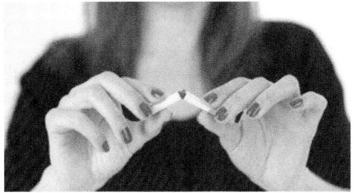

If you have diabetes, you already have an increased chance of developing cardiovascular disease, such as a heart attack, stroke or circulatory problems in the legs.

Combine this with smoking (which can also double your risk of complications) and you make the chances of developing these diseases even higher.

Giving up can be hard, but you don't have to carry the burden of quitting on your own. It has been shown that you are more likely to quit if you get the right support. Whichever method you choose, there are clear benefits from quitting and plenty of support to help you.

Chapter 5:
Prediabetes

Prediabetes means that your blood sugar level is higher than normal but not yet high enough to be classified as type 2 diabetes. Without intervention, prediabetes is likely to become type 2 diabetes in 10 years or less. If you have prediabetes, the long-term damage of diabetes — especially to your heart and circulatory system — may already be starting.

There's good news, however. Prediabetes can be an opportunity for you to improve your health. Progression from prediabetes to type 2 diabetes isn't inevitable.

With healthy lifestyle changes — such as eating healthy foods, including physical activity in your daily routine and maintaining a healthy weight — you may be able to bring your blood sugar level back to normal.

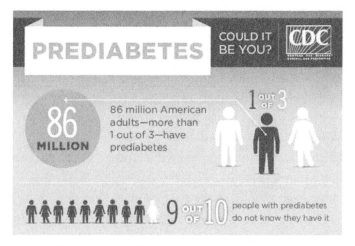

In pre-diabetes, blood sugar levels are slightly higher than normal, but still not as high as in diabetes. If diabetes is "runaway blood sugar" think of pre-diabetes as blood sugar that is "halfway out the door."

People almost always develop pre-diabetes before they get type 2 diabetes. The rise in blood sugar levels that is seen in pre-diabetes starts when the body begins to develop a problem called "**insulin** resistance." Insulin is an important hormone that helps you to process **glucose** (blood sugar). If usual amounts of insulin can't trigger the body to move **glucose** out of the bloodstream and into your cells, then you have insulin resistance.

Once insulin resistance begins, it can worsen over time. When you have pre-diabetes, you make extra insulin to keep your sugar levels near to normal. Insulin resistance can worsen as you age, and it worsens with weight gain. If your insulin resistance progresses, eventually you can't compensate well enough by making extra insulin. When this occurs, your sugar levels will increase, and you will have diabetes.

Depending on what a blood sugar test finds, pre-diabetes can be more specifically called "impaired glucose (sugar) tolerance" or "impaired fasting glucose." Impaired fasting glucose means that blood sugar increase after you haven't eaten for a while – for example, in the morning, before breakfast.

Impaired glucose tolerance means that blood sugar levels reach a surprisingly high level after you eat sugar. To diagnose impaired glucose tolerance, doctors usually use what is called a "glucose tolerance test." For this test you drink a sugary solution, and then you have blood drawn after a short time.

Having pre-diabetes does not automatically mean you will get diabetes, but it does put you at an increased risk. Pre-diabetes is also a risk factor for heart disease. Like people with type 2 diabetes, those with pre-diabetes tend to be overweight, have high blood pressure and have unhealthy cholesterol levels.

Symptoms

Pre-diabetes is often called a "silent" condition because it usually has no symptoms. You can have pre-diabetes for several years without knowing it. Certain risk factors increase the chance that you have pre-diabetes. These risk factors include:

- Being overweight
- Being 45 years or older
- A family history of diabetes
- Low levels of high-density lipoprotein (HDL) cholesterol (the "good" cholesterol)
- High triglycerides
- High blood pressure
- A history of gestational diabetes
- Being African-American, American Indian, Asian-American, Pacific Islander or Hispanic American/Latino

If you have one or more of these risk factors, your doctor may recommend a blood sugar test. An abnormal result is likely to be the first sign that you have pre-diabetes.

Diagnosis

The same blood sugar tests that are used for diabetes are used to diagnose pre-diabetes. For diagnosing pre-diabetes, your doctor can order one of the following:

- A fasting blood glucose test
- An oral glucose tolerance test
- A hemoglobin A1C (HbA1C) blood test

In a fasting glucose test, blood sugar levels are measured after at least eight hours of not eating. Most people prefer to have the test done the morning after fasting overnight.

In the oral glucose tolerance test, blood sugar levels are first measured after an overnight fast. You then drink a sugary solution, and two hours later another blood sample is drawn. This second test is known as a "glucose challenge." In healthy people, the glucose challenge will cause blood sugar levels to rise slightly and fall quickly. In someone with pre-diabetes or diabetes, these levels rise very high or fall slowly, so they will be abnormally high during the two-hour blood test.

A hemoglobin A1C blood test can be done at any time during the day. It does not require fasting. The result reflects an average of your blood sugar over the preceding 3 months.

Here is how to interpret the results of these tests (mg/dL = milligrams per deciliter):

Fasting glucose test
- Normal – Below 100 mg/dL
- Pre-diabetes – Between 100 and 125 mg/dL
- Diabetes – 126 mg/dL or higher

Oral glucose tolerance test
- Normal – Below 140 mg/dL
- Pre-diabetes – Between 140 mg/dL and 199 mg/dL
- Diabetes – 200 mg/dL or higher

Hemoglobin A1C test
- Normal – 5.6% or below
- Pre-diabetes – Between 5.7% and 6.4%
- Diabetes – 6.5% or higher

Expected Duration

Pre-diabetes sugar levels can remain slightly above normal, can return to normal, or can increase to a range that leads to a diagnosis of diabetes. As many as 1 in 10 people with impaired glucose tolerance will develop diabetes within one year. What happens to your pre-diabetes depends on whether you are able to prevent insulin resistance from progressing. If insulin resistance is kept in check, pre-diabetes may never become diabetes. If you do not adjust your lifestyle to increase exercise and improve diet, blood sugar levels will probably eventually rise to diabetic levels. Once this happens, medication is usually required to bring your blood sugar back to near-normal levels.

Prevention

It surprises many people to learn that they may be able to prevent pre-diabetes and diabetes. To reduce your risk of both pre-diabetes and diabetes:

- Maintain an ideal body weight. Aim for a body mass index (BMI) between 18.5 and 25.
- Exercise regularly. Both aerobic and strengthening exercises can reduce blood sugar. You should exercise for a minimum of 30 minutes daily.
- Eat a balanced diet with just enough calories to maintain a healthy weight.

If you are overweight, aim to lose weight. Even modest weight loss of 10 or 15 pounds in a person who is 200 pounds can dramatically reduce the risk of diabetes.

Treatment

The purpose for treating pre-diabetes is to prevent diabetes from setting in. The same measures recommended for preventing pre-diabetes (see above) work for treating it, too.

The most effective treatment for pre-diabetes is to lose weight and exercise at least 30 minutes a day. Weight loss and exercise can improve insulin resistance and can lower elevated blood sugar levels so that you don't progress to develop diabetes.

Additionally, the drug **metformin** (**Glucophage**) can lower the risk of getting diabetes, and it can add to the benefits of weight loss and exercise. Check with your doctor about whether taking metformin to prevent diabetes is a good idea for you. If your doctor feels that you have an especially high risk for progressing to diabetes, you may want to consider preventive treatment with this medication.

When To Call a Professional

It's best to have annual glucose tests to monitor pre-diabetes. Also, look for symptoms that can suggest the development of new diabetes, such as:

- Excessive urination, thirst and hunger
- Unexplained weight loss
- Increased susceptibility to infections, especially yeast or fungal infections of the skin and vagina
- Confused thinking, weakness or nausea.

Chapter 6:
Diagnosis

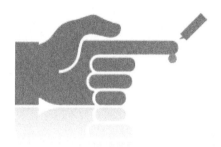

Blood tests are used to diagnosis diabetes and prediabetes because early in the disease type 2 diabetes may have no symptoms. All diabetes blood tests involve drawing blood at a health care provider's office or commercial facility and sending the sample to a lab for analysis. Lab analysis of blood is needed to ensure test results are accurate. Glucose measuring devices used in a health care provider's office, such as finger-stick devices, are not accurate enough for diagnosis but may be used as a quick indicator of high blood glucose.

Testing enables health care providers to find and treat diabetes before complications occur and to find and treat prediabetes, which can delay or prevent type 2 diabetes from developing.

Any one of the following tests can be used for diagnosis:

- an **A1C** test, also called the hemoglobin A1c, HbA1c, or glycohemoglobin test

- a **fasting plasma glucose (FPG)** test
- an **oral glucose tolerance test (OGTT)**

*Not all tests are recommended for diagnosing all types of diabetes. See the individual test descriptions for details.

Another blood test, the random plasma glucose (RPG) test, is sometimes used to diagnose diabetes during a regular health checkup. If the RPG measures 200 micrograms per deciliter or above, and the individual also shows symptoms of diabetes, then a health care provider may diagnose diabetes.

Symptoms of diabetes include

- increased urination
- increased thirst
- unexplained weight loss

Other symptoms can include fatigue, blurred vision, increased hunger, and sores that do not heal.

Any test used to diagnose diabetes requires confirmation with a second measurement unless clear symptoms of diabetes exist.

The following table provides the blood test levels for diagnosis of diabetes for nonpregnant adults and diagnosis of prediabetes.

Blood Test Levels for Diagnosis of Diabetes and Prediabetes

	A1C (percent)	Fasting Plasma Glucose (mg/dL)	Oral Glucose Tolerance Test (mg/dL)
Diabetes	6.5 or above	126 or above	200 or above
Prediabetes	5.7 to 6.4	100 to 125	140 to 199
Normal	About 5	99 or below	139 or below

Definitions: mg = milligram, dL = deciliter
For all three tests, within the prediabetes range, the higher the test result, the greater the risk of diabetes.

A1C Test

The A1C test is used to detect type 2 diabetes and prediabetes but is not recommended for diagnosis of type 1 diabetes or gestational diabetes. The A1C test is a blood test that reflects the average of a person's blood glucose levels over the past 3 months and does not show daily fluctuations. The A1C test is more convenient for patients than the traditional glucose tests because it does not require fasting and can be performed at any time of the day.

The A1C test result is reported as a percentage. The higher the percentage, the higher a person's blood glucose levels have been. A normal A1C level is below 5.7 percent.

An A1C of 5.7 to 6.4 percent indicates prediabetes.

People diagnosed with prediabetes may be retested in 1 year. People with an A1C below 5.7 percent may still be at risk for diabetes, depending on the presence of other characteristics that put them at risk, also known as risk factors. People with an A1C above 6.0 percent should be considered at very high risk of developing diabetes. A level of 6.5 percent or above means a person has diabetes.

Laboratory analysis. When the A1C test is used for diagnosis, the blood sample must be sent to a laboratory using a method that is certified by the NGSP to ensure the results are standardized. Blood samples analyzed in a health care provider's office, known as point-of-care tests, are not standardized for diagnosing diabetes.

Abnormal results. The A1C test can be unreliable for diagnosing or monitoring diabetes in people with certain conditions known to interfere with the results. Interference should be suspected when A1C results seem very different from the results of a blood glucose test. People of African, Mediterranean, or Southeast Asian descent or people with family members with sickle cell anemia or a thalassemia are particularly at risk of interference.

False A1C test results may also occur in people with other problems that affect their blood or hemoglobin such as chronic kidney disease, liver disease, or anemia.

Changes in Diagnostic Testing

In the past, the A1C test was used to monitor blood glucose levels but not for diagnosis. The A1C test has now been standardized, and in 2009, an international expert committee recommended it be used for diagnosis of type 2 diabetes and prediabetes.[2]

Fasting Plasma Glucose Test

The FPG test is used to detect diabetes and prediabetes. The FPG test has been the most common test used for diagnosing diabetes because it is more convenient than the OGTT and less expensive. The FPG test measures blood glucose in a person who has fasted for at least 8 hours and is most reliable when given in the morning.

People with a fasting glucose level of 100 to 125 mg/dL have impaired fasting glucose (IFG), or prediabetes. A level of 126 mg/dL or above, confirmed by repeating the test on another day, means a person has diabetes.

Oral Glucose Tolerance Test

The OGTT can be used to diagnose diabetes, prediabetes, and gestational diabetes. Research has shown that the OGTT is more sensitive than the FPG test, but it is less convenient to administer. When used to test for diabetes or prediabetes, the OGTT measures blood glucose after a person fasts for at least 8 hours and 2 hours after the person drinks a liquid containing 75 grams of glucose dissolved in water.

If the 2-hour blood glucose level is between 140 and 199 mg/dL, the person has a type of prediabetes called impaired glucose tolerance (IGT). If confirmed by a second test, a 2-hour glucose level of 200 mg/dL or above means a person has diabetes.

Are diabetes blood test results always accurate?

All laboratory test results can vary from day to day and from test to test. Results can vary

- **within the person being tested.** A person's blood glucose levels normally move up and down depending on meals, exercise, sickness, and stress.
- **between different tests.** Each test measures blood glucose levels in a different way.
- **within the same test.** Even when the same blood sample is repeatedly measured in the same laboratory, the results may vary due to small changes in temperature, equipment, or sample handling.

Although all these tests can be used to indicate diabetes, in some people one test will indicate a diagnosis of diabetes when another test does not. People with differing test results may be in an early stage of the disease, where blood glucose levels have not risen high enough to show on every test.

Health care providers take all these variations into account when considering test results and repeat laboratory tests for confirmation. Diabetes develops over time, so even with variations in test results, health care providers can tell when overall blood glucose levels are becoming too high.

Chapter 7:
Prevention

Diabetes prevention is as basic as eating more healthfully, becoming more physically active and losing a few extra pounds — and it's never too late to start. Making a few simple changes in your lifestyle now may help you avoid the serious health complications of diabetes down the road, such as nerve, kidney and heart damage. Consider the latest diabetes prevention tips from the American Diabetes Association.

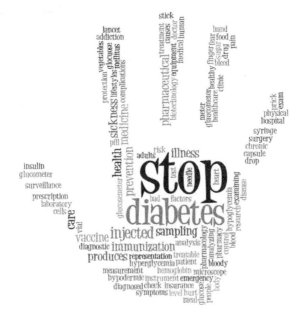

Tip 1: Get more physical activity
There are many benefits to regular physical activity. Exercise can help you:

- Lose weight
- Lower your blood sugar
- Boost your sensitivity to insulin — which helps keep your blood sugar within a normal range

Research shows that both aerobic exercise and resistance training can help control diabetes, but the greater benefit comes from a fitness program that includes both.

Tip 2: Get plenty of fiber
It's rough, it's tough — and it may help you:

- Reduce your risk of diabetes by improving your blood sugar control
- Lower your risk of heart disease
- Promote weight loss by helping you feel full

Foods high in fiber include fruits, vegetables, beans, whole grains, nuts and seeds.

Tip 3: Go for whole grains
Although it's not clear why, whole grains may reduce your risk of diabetes and help maintain blood sugar levels. Try to make at least half your grains whole grains. Many foods made from whole grains come ready to eat, including various breads, pasta products and many cereals. Look for the word "whole" on the package and among the first few items in the ingredient list.

Tip 4: Lose extra weight

If you're overweight, diabetes prevention may hinge on weight loss. Every pound you lose can improve your health, and you may be surprised by how much. Participants in one large study who lost a modest amount of weight — around 7 percent of initial body weight — and exercised regularly reduced the risk of developing diabetes by almost 60 percent.

Tip 5: Skip fad diets and just make healthier choices

Low-carb diets, the glycemic index diet or other fad diets may help you lose weight at first, but their effectiveness at preventing diabetes isn't known nor are their long-term effects. And by excluding or strictly limiting a particular food group, you may be giving up essential nutrients. Instead, think variety and portion control as part of an overall healthy-eating plan.

When to see your doctor

If you're older than age 45 and your weight is normal, ask your doctor if diabetes testing is appropriate for you. The American Diabetes Association recommends blood glucose screening if:

- You're age 45 or older and overweight
- You're younger than age 45 and overweight with one or more additional risk factors for type 2 diabetes — such as a sedentary lifestyle or a family history of diabetes

Share your concerns about diabetes prevention with

your doctor. He or she will applaud your efforts to keep diabetes at bay, and perhaps offer additional suggestions based on your medical history or other factors.

Chapter 8:
Treatment

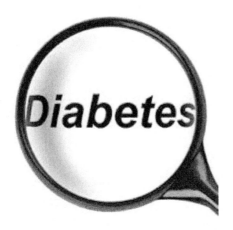

The basic aim of diabetes treatment is to reduce risk of complications by reducing cardiovascular risk factors, such as smoking, poor diet, lack of exercise, high blood pressure and high cholesterol, and to keep blood glucose as normal as possible.

Diabetes treatment should also involve measures to reduce this risk.

Your treatment plan

Treatment for diabetes depends on the individual.

All people with diabetes should attend 'structured education', which enables you to understand how to manage your diabetes day by day.

It starts the first time you give yourself an insulin injection or take a diabetes tablet, and it continues through eating a well-balanced diet and starting an exercise programme.

To help you get the most out of treatment, consult your diabetes health professional, which may include your GP, practice nurse or hospital healthcare team.

Diet and exercise

Diet and exercise can help all types of diabetes, but have a direct effect on controllingtype 2 diabetes.

A special diet used to be recommended for diabetes.

It's now believed a normal well-balanced diet is best for diabetes. The principles of healthy eating are:

- eat regular meals (to prevent dips and spikes in blood sugar)
- cut down on high sugar foods
- reduce fat intake
- cut down on salt
- eat at least five portions of fruit and vegetables a day

If you're overweight, go on a calorie-controlled diet to lose pounds.

This is because being overweight further increases your higher risk of cardiovascular disease – think of weight loss as a necessary part of your treatment.

Regular exercise helps all types of diabetes and provides many benefits, including reducing your risk of cardiovascular disease.

You should aim to do moderate exercise (such as a brisk walk) for at least 30 minutes on most days of the week.

Many people with type 2 diabetes are overweight and find it difficult to lose weight.

If diet and exercise don't produce sufficient weight loss, your doctor may consider prescribing an anti-obesity medicine.

Xenical (orlistat) is currently the only medicine available on prescription in the UK for treating obesity.

Reducing cardiovascular risk

As well as diet and exercise, you can reduce your risk of cardiovascular disease by:

- stopping smoking
- lowering blood pressure
- lowering body weight.
- lowering cholesterol
- taking medicines called statins.

Statins are used to lower cholesterol levels.

Recent studies have shown they may also reduce the risk of cardiovascular events, such as strokes and heart attacks, regardless of whether you have a high or low level of cholesterol.

Insulin treatment

For people with type 1 diabetes, and some with type 2 diabetes, insulin treatment is needed to increase the insulin level in the blood and bring down the blood glucose level.

There are various types of insulin available:

- those that act quickly and last for a short time
- those that act more slowly and provide a background control of blood glucose throughout the day.

There are also combinations of these that come pre-mixed.

The aim is to mimic the body's natural production of insulin so that blood sugar is controlled, without it falling too low (hypoglycaemia).

This is done through the timing of doses and by using a combination of insulin preparations that are absorbed at different rates.

The amount of insulin used needs to be balanced against the amount you eat and how much exercise you do.

At the start, insulin treatment may seem quite daunting, but it soon becomes a simple process. Your diabetes team are always there to advise you.

Insulin can't be taken by mouth because the digestive enzymes in the gut break it down. Oral insulin is presently being researched but it is not available for routine clinical use.

Various other delivery techniques are still under investigation.

Insulin infusion pumps are becoming more commonly used. A short-acting insulin is delivered by a small pump into the fatty subcutaneous tissue under the skin, called the continuous subcutaneous insulin infusion (CSII).

These pumps are expensive but are available on prescription to certain people with type 1 diabetes and difficulties with diabetes control or hypoglycaemia unawareness. Specialist hospital clinics supervise this treatment.

The insulin is pumped into a small plastic tube with a small needle at the end which is injected under the skin. Less injections are required as the needle only needs to be changed every two days.

CSII is especially useful in children or type 1 diabetic patients of any age who have problems with hypoglycaemia (low blood sugar) or cannot get satisfactory blood sugar control with standard injections.

Treatments for type 2 diabetes

People with type 2 diabetes whose blood sugar is not controlled sufficiently by diet and exercise will be prescribed oral medication to help lower their blood sugar.

However, oral treatment shouldn't replace diet and exercise, which are still an essential part of treatment.

There are various different types of oral medication for treating type 2 diabetes:

- some increase the amount of insulin secreted by the pancreas, eg sulfonylureas such as gliclazide, as well as the newer medicines nateglinide and repaglinide

- some increase the action of insulin in the body, ie they reduce insulin resistance, egmetformin and glitazones such as pioglitazone
- some delay the absorption of glucose from the digestive system, eg acarbose
- some increase insulin secretion and reduce glucagon secretion, eg gliptins such as assitagliptin, linagliptin, saxagliptin and vildaglipti n
- some allow excess glucose to be excreted in the urine, eg dapagliflozin andcanagliflozin
- there are also injectable medicines for type 2 diabetes that work by increasing insulin secretion, reducing glucagon secretion and slowing down the passage of food from the stomach into the intestine. These include exenatide, liraglutide and lixisenatide.

The type of medicine initially used depends mainly on whether you are overweight.

- Metformin is usually the medicine of first choice for people who are overweight, because it doesn't cause weight gain.
- People who are not overweight will usually be prescribed a sulfonylurea, such as gliclazide, as the first choice.

If the first medicine does not reduce blood sugar sufficiently, another type can be added to treatment. This is called combination therapy. Sometimes three different medicines may be needed.

Chapter 9:
Blood Glucose Monitoring

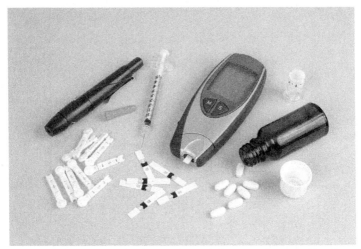

Measuring blood glucose levels tells you how effective your treatment is at keeping your blood sugar as close to normal as possible.

People on insulin should check blood glucose levels regularly, but those on diet only or tablets do not need to check blood glucose levels.

There are no hard and fast rules for how often you should test.

- Some people feel monitoring their blood sugar regularly gives them more control, particularly if they adjust their insulin dose or make changes to their diet and exercise levels on the basis of the results.

- Other people find frequent monitoring makes them anxious.

- You should decide how often to test your blood glucose in conjunction with your diabetes team.

- Your tests should give you a picture of how your blood glucose fluctuates throughout the day, from day to day.

- This means your tests will be more helpful if you take them at different times of day, and on days when you've done different levels of activity.

- The most useful times to measure blood glucose are fasting (before breakfast), just before meals, around two hours after meals and before bed.

- You should test your blood glucose level when you feel unwell. You may need to test your blood glucose more frequently during pregnancy.

- Measuring the amount of a compound called glycated haemoglobin (HbA1c) in the blood is also helpful for monitoring diabetes treatment.

- It provides a measure of the average glucose level over the previous couple of months and gives a better idea of whether your treatment is adequate.

Your body uses the sugar, also known as glucose, in the foods you eat for energy. Think of it as a fuel that keeps your body moving throughout the day.

Blood Sugar Highs and Lows

Type 2 diabetes decreases the body's production of insulin, which is a hormone that regulates blood sugar. Without enough insulin, sugar builds up in the blood and can damage nerves and blood vessels. This increase of blood sugar also increases your risk for heart disease and stroke. Over time, high blood sugar, also known as hyperglycemia, can lead to more health problems, including kidney failure and blindness.

"Keeping blood sugar stable can help prevent the long-term consequences of fluctuations," says Melissa Li-Ng, MD, an endocrinologist at the Cleveland Clinic in Ohio. Dr. Li-Ng explains that high blood sugar can cause a number of symptoms that include:

- Fatigue
- Increased thirst
- Blurry vision
- Frequent urination

On the flip side, if you're not closely monitoring your blood sugar levels, they can drop too low. Warning signs of low blood sugar, or hypoglycemia, include:

- Dizziness
- Irritability
- Sweating
- Weakness
- Lack of coordination

Keeping Your Blood Sugar Steady

With certain strategies, you can help prevent spikes in your blood sugar levels, says Toby Smithson, RD, LDN, CDE,a spokesperson for the Academy of Nutrition and Dietetics and the founder of DiabetesEveryday.com.

Rather than focus on things you shouldn't have, try incorporating the following foods and healthy habits into your daily type 2 diabetes routine:

1. **Go nuts.** Nuts such as almonds, walnuts, and pistachios contain healthy fat that slows the body's absorption of sugar. But be sure to limit how many nuts you eat in one sitting because even healthy fats contain calories, Smithson says. Just six almonds or four pecan halves have the same number of calories as one teaspoon of butter.

2. **Eat whole grains.** Oat bran, barley, and rye are fiber-rich foods that contain beta-glucan. This soluble fiber increases the amount of time it takes for your stomach to empty after eating and prevents spikes in blood sugar. Remember, though, that these foods are still carbohydrates. "Whole grains will still raise your blood sugar, just not as quickly and as high as processed foods," Li-Ng says.

3. **Veg out.** Packed with fiber, non-starchy vegetables such as broccoli, cucumber, and carrots can also help prevent surges in blood sugar levels while providing essential nutrients.

4. **Spice up with cinnamon.** Cinnamon may do more than just add flavor to foods. A 2013 study published in the journal Annals of Family Medicine showed that cinnamon is linked to a significant drop in fasting blood sugar levels. Cinnamon may stimulate insulin secretions from the pancreas," Li-Ng says. Although more research is needed, Smithson says there's no reason why people with type 2 diabetes shouldn't try to add cinnamon in their diets.

5. **Be versatile with vinegar.** A 2012 study published in the Journal of Community Hospital Internal Medicine Perspectives suggested that vinegar could help slow the absorption of sugar by the body. The research revealed that 2 ounces of apple cider vinegar improved fasting blood sugar levels and insulin sensitivity. Although the potential health benefits of vinegar are still being investigated, Li-Ng often advises people with type 2 diabetes to take 1 tablespoon of vinegar with each meal, saying that any type of vinegar is good.

6. **Don't skip meals.** It's important to spread out your daily food intake, starting with breakfast. Consuming more food in just one or two meals a day causes greater fluctuations in blood sugar levels, Li-Ng says. "Three healthy meals a day with two nutritious snacks in between can help maintain stable blood sugar," she says.

7. **Don't drink on an empty stomach.** If you haven't eaten, drinking alcohol can cause your blood sugar to drop up to 24 hours later. This happens because the body is working to get rid of it. If you want to drink alcohol, check your blood sugar first. It's also important to eat before or while you drink. Another caution: Smithson says that symptoms of low blood sugar, such as slurred speech and dizziness, could be mistaken for drunkenness.

8. **Plan ahead.** Anticipate the unexpected and carry healthy snacks that can prevent your blood sugar level from dropping too low. Smithson recommends carrying granola bars with you as well as some quick-acting glucose tablets, also known as "sugar pills."

DISCLAIMER AND/OR LEGAL NOTICES: Every effort has been made to accurately represent this book and it's potential. Results vary with every individual, and your results may or may not be different from those depicted. No promises, guarantees or warranties, whether stated or implied, have been made that you will produce any specific result from this book. Your efforts are individual and unique, and may vary from those shown. Your success depends on your efforts, background and motivation.

The material in this publication is provided for educational and informational purposes only and is not intended as medical advice. The information contained in this book should not be used to diagnose or treat any illness, metabolic disorder, disease or health problem. Always consult your physician or health care provider before beginning any nutrition or exercise program. Use of the programs, advice, and information contained in this book is at the sole choice and risk of the reader.

Printed in Great Britain
by Amazon

56769843R00041